Essential Oils: Essential Introductory Beginners Guide - How To Use Essential Oils For Optimal Physical And Emotional Health And Beauty. With 16 Recipes included

by Katey Lyon

Disclaimer

The information contained in this book is for educational and informational purposes only. It is not intended to diagnose, treat, cure, or prevent any disease. Always consult with a qualified healthcare professional before using essential oils, especially if you are pregnant, nursing, taking medication, or have a medical condition.

The author and publisher assume no responsibility for any adverse effects or consequences resulting from the use of the information contained in this book.

Permitted Use

This book is licensed for personal, non-commercial use only. The author and publisher assume no responsibility for any adverse effects or consequences resulting from the use of the information contained in this book.

This book is licensed for personal, non-commercial use only.

Table of Contents

Chapter 1: Introduction To Essential Oils

Introduction

My interest in essential oils began a few years ago when my puppy had to undergo surgery. She was only six months old and needed to be spayed. After the procedure, she was behaving normally, but we had to take special care of her wound and try to keep her calm so she could recover properly.

I did not want to rely heavily on medication because she was still very young, so I decided to try something natural. I had heard that lavender essential oil could help promote relaxation and calmness. I prepared a simple spray with lavender and lightly sprayed it around the house. I also applied a very small amount near her ears. The effect was remarkable. She remained calm and relaxed, which helped her recover comfortably.

This experience sparked my curiosity. I wanted to learn more about essential oils and how they could be used in everyday life. Soon after, I took an introductory aromatherapy course and discovered that essential oils have been used for centuries to support physical health, emotional well-being, and beauty.

Why Essential Oils Have Become So Popular

In recent years, essential oils have gained significant global popularity. Many people are looking for natural ways to support their health and reduce stress in their daily lives. As a result, aromatherapy has become an important part of holistic wellness practices.

Essential oils are concentrated extracts obtained from plants such as flowers, leaves, bark, roots, and fruits. These extracts capture the plant's natural aroma and beneficial properties. Because they are derived from nature, many people prefer them as a complementary option to support their well-being.

The increasing interest in natural remedies, self-care, and holistic health has led more people to explore the benefits of essential oils. Today, they are commonly used in homes, spas, wellness centers, and even healthcare environments.

How Aromatherapy Is Used Today

Aromatherapy is the practice of using essential oils to support physical and emotional well-being. Essential oils can be used in several ways, including inhalation, massage, baths, and diffusers.

Many people use essential oils to help promote relaxation, improve sleep, reduce stress, and create a pleasant environment at home. Others use them as part of skincare routines, massage therapy, or natural home care products.

For example, lavender is commonly used to promote relaxation and better sleep. Peppermint is often used to help relieve headaches and increase alertness. Lemon and orange oils are popular for creating uplifting and refreshing environments.

When used properly and safely, essential oils can become a valuable addition to everyday wellness routines.

Benefits of Natural Remedies

Natural remedies have been used for thousands of years in traditional healing practices across many cultures. Plants, herbs, and natural extracts have long been valued for their potential to support health and balance in the body.

One advantage of natural remedies, such as essential oils, is that they can be incorporated into daily life in simple ways. Many people enjoy using them to create relaxing environments, support emotional balance, or enhance personal care routines.

It is important to remember that aromatherapy is considered a complementary approach to wellness. Essential oils are not meant to replace professional medical care but can be used alongside healthy lifestyle choices to support overall well-being.

What You Will Learn in This Book

This beginner's guide is designed to introduce you to the world of essential oils and help you understand how they can be used safely and effectively.

- What essential oils are and how they are produced
- The basics of aromatherapy
- How essential oils interact with the body
- Safe methods for using essential oils
- The role of carrier oils in aromatherapy
- Essential oils that support health, emotional balance, and beauty
- Simple recipes you can prepare at home

Whether you are completely new to essential oils or simply curious about their benefits, this book will provide a clear and practical introduction to help you begin your aromatherapy journey.

Chapter 2: Understanding Essential Oils

What Are Essential Oils

Essential oils are plant extracts that have been created by steam distillation of plant material from a single botanical source. The essential oil is separated from the condensed steam, and nothing is added or taken away.

These plants contain therapeutic properties known to help with some health ailments. Such essential oils are used in clinical aromatherapy practice to help with physical problems (pain, arthritis, nausea, etc.), emotional problems (depression, anxiety, stress, etc.), skin care, weight loss and much more.

Both organic and non-organic essential oils have the same therapeutic properties because both are extracted from plants.

What is Aromatherapy

Aromatherapy is a therapy that uses essential oils and water-based colloids obtained from plant materials to promote physical, emotional and spiritual health and balance. According to the Canadian Federation of Aromatherapist, aromatherapy is the art and science of using essential oils for improving and maintaining health and beauty.

The actual word is "Aroatherapie," which was created in 1928 by Rene Murice Gattefosse, a French chemist while he was conducting an experiment. His hands were severely burned in a lab explosion, and he found that Lavender healed them.

How Essential Oils Work

According to Deepak Chopra, a Medical Doctor and leading international spiritual Guru, he explains that when you inhale a scent, the aroma travels directly to the hypothalamus. The hypothalamus is an organ in the brain responsible for regulating growth, sleep, emotional responses, and more.

This aroma flows through the body's limbic system and into an area of the hippocampus; that is the part of the brain that's responsible for memory. This process is called neuro-associative conditioning, which is the body's ability to link a healing response to a particular smell.

The sense of smell connects you directly with your emotions, instincts, and memories. Studies performed by NYU Langone Medical Center concluded that when specific aromas were inhaled through the nose, the symptoms of headaches, menstrual pain, and respiratory infection subsided.

Another study performed by the University of Maryland Medical Center concluded that inhaling lavender, rose, and frankincense alleviated anxiety, stress, and depression. Also, the use of peppermint subsided nausea and chamomile subsided the pain.

Essential oils follow three main pathways to gain entry to the body: inhalation, ingestion, and absorption through the skin.

Inhalation

Inhalation is the access via the nasal passages; it is usually the quickest efficient route in the treatment of emotional problems such as stress and depression. This is because the nose has direct contact with the brain, which is responsible for triggering the effects of essential oils. Methods of inhalation include:

The use of tissues that contain 5 to 6 drops of essential oil placed inside the shirt, blouse, or nightwear.

Hands. This is an excellent method, but it should be confined to emergencies only and isn't suitable for children.

Put 1 drop in your palm, rub both hands, and place the hands over your nose, avoiding the eyes, then take a deep nasal breath.
Bath. Putting essential oils into the tub is effective because not only do they come into gentle contact with the skin, but they are also inhaled at the same time. This is a double benefit.
Spray bottle. A quick way of freshening the air, it can be used in the house, car or by spraying yourself.
Diffusers and Vaporizers: The main difference between diffusers and vaporizers is that diffusers push all the

essential oil molecules out at the same time, while vaporizers push the lightest essential oil molecules out first.

Steam Inhalation: You can fill a bowl with warm water and add a few drops, cover your head with a towel and inhale the aroma for around five minutes.

Candles: A true aromatherapy candle is made with pure essential oils and is made from beeswax or soy.

Ingestion

When essential oils are taken by mouth, knowledge of the ingredients of the essential oils is of paramount importance. This means it is essential to know the strength of concentration, the nature of any diluents used, and the length of time for which it is to be taken.

Most aroma therapists are cautious about using ingestion because of the greater danger of an excessive dose reaching the liver than if done by external application.

Absorption via the skin

Massage: This is the best way to induce deep relaxation, release tension, improve circulation to the muscles and release suppressed feelings.

Compress: This is the best way to use essential oils when you have pain or inflammation in the body. Fill a bowl with warm water, add a few drops of appropriate essential oil, and soak a face cloth, squeeze the access water out and apply the compress to the affected area.

Chapter 3: Safe Use of Essential Oils

Cautions And Tips When Using Essential Oils

Be cautious of using essential oils during pregnancy, with children, and babies. Always check the dosage and always consult a health practitioner. It is also important to be careful with the use of essential oils in certain medical conditions.

For example, if you have allergies and sensitive skin, avoid the use of peppermint and clove. With high blood pressure, avoid using sage, and if you are suffering from diabetes, use extra caution.

If you are taking medications or you are under treatment, especially with homeopathy, be cautious and always consult your health practitioner. The following is a list of other general precautions for the use of essential oils:
Avoid contact with the eyes, nose, and lips.

Essential oils must be stored in dark, glass bottles.
Always dilute essential oils with a carrier oil before applying to the skin.

Keep essential oils in bottles out of reach of children, babies and pets.

Discontinue the use of essential oils if irritation occurs. People who suffer from allergies to perfumes or asthma need to be cautious.

Use in low concentration when dealing with babies, children, pets, pregnancy, elderly people, or those with a serious illness.
Keep essential oils away from the heat and flames.

What Are Carrier Oils?

Carrier oils, also known as base oil or vegetable oil, constitute the bulk of the material used in an aromatherapy massage. Their function is to carry or act as a vehicle for administering the essential oils to the body and also as lubricants to make massage movements possible.

Some carrier oils are jojoba oil, olive oil, grape seed oil, rose hip oil, etc. Let's see some benefits of the most well-known types.

Sweet almond oil is one of the most popular carrier oils. The advantage over others is that it has less of a tendency to become rancid. This oil is used in laxative preparations and is an excellent emollient, and it also nourishes dry skin and helps soothe inflammation.

Rapeseed is a gentle emollient and leaves the skin with a smooth satiny finish without feeling greasy.
Avocado oil has anti-wrinkle properties, is a moisturizing and is recommended for dry skins.

Jojoba oil contains the anti-inflammatory agent myristic acid, making it beneficial for arthritis and rheumatism. It is used for acne, sunburn, and eczema.

Rose Hip possesses therapeutic properties and has an effect on the skin to minimize premature aging and wrinkles, and it is also helpful for wounds, burns, and eczema.

Carrier Oils Guide

Carrier oils play an important role in aromatherapy. Because essential oils are highly concentrated, they should usually be diluted before applying them to the skin. Carrier oils help reduce the strength of essential oils and allow them to be safely absorbed by the skin.

Most carrier oils are derived from nuts, seeds, or plants. They often contain vitamins, antioxidants, and nourishing fatty acids that benefit the skin.

Below are some of the most commonly used carrier oils in aromatherapy.

Jojoba Oil
Jojoba oil is one of the most popular carrier oils used in aromatherapy. Technically, it is not an oil but a liquid wax extracted from the seeds of the jojoba plant.

Benefits
Jojoba oil closely resembles the skin's natural oils, which allows it to absorb easily without leaving a greasy feeling. It is rich in vitamins and antioxidants that support healthy

skin.

Common Uses
Jojoba oil is frequently used in facial serums, massage oils, and skincare blends. It works well for both dry and oily skin types.

Best For

- Facial care
- Acne treatments
- Anti-aging blends

Sweet Almond Oil
Sweet almond oil is a light, nourishing carrier oil extracted from almonds. It has been used in skincare for centuries.

Benefits
This oil is rich in vitamin E and fatty acids that help moisturize and soften the skin.

Common Uses
Sweet almond oil is often used in massage blends and body oils because it spreads easily across the skin.

Best For

- Massage oils
- Body moisturizers
- Dry skin care

Coconut Oil
Coconut oil is widely used as both a cooking oil and a carrier oil. It is extracted from the meat of coconuts.

Benefits
Coconut oil has moisturizing properties and helps protect the skin. Fractionated coconut oil is often preferred in aromatherapy because it remains liquid and absorbs easily.

Common Uses
It is commonly used in massage oils, skincare products, and hair treatments.

Best For

- Body oils
- Hair care treatments
- Moisturizing blends

Grapeseed Oil
Grapeseed oil is extracted from the seeds of grapes. It has a very light texture and absorbs quickly into the skin.

Benefits
Grapeseed oil is rich in antioxidants and essential fatty acids that support healthy skin.

Common Uses
Because it is light and non-greasy, grapeseed oil is often used in facial oils and massage blends.

Best For

- Oily skin
- Massage blends
- Light skincare formulas

Olive Oil

Olive oil has been used for thousands of years in skincare and traditional medicine. It is extracted from olives and contains many beneficial nutrients.

Benefits
Olive oil is rich in antioxidants and vitamin E, which help nourish and protect the skin.

Common Uses
It is often used in massage oils and homemade skincare recipes.

Best For

- Dry skin
- Body oils
- Homemade beauty treatments

Argan Oil
Argan oil is extracted from the kernels of the argan tree, which grows mainly in Morocco.

Benefits
Argan oil is rich in vitamin E and essential fatty acids. It is widely used in cosmetic products because it helps hydrate and nourish the skin and hair.

Common Uses
Argan oil is often used in facial serums, hair treatments, and anti-aging skincare blends.

Best For

- Hair treatments
- Anti-aging skincare

- Dry skin care

Choosing the Right Carrier Oil

When selecting a carrier oil, consider your skin type and how you plan to use the blend.
For example:

- **Light oils** like grapeseed are ideal for facial care.
- **Nourishing oils** like sweet almond or olive oil work well for massage.
- **Specialty oils** like argan oil are excellent for hair and skin treatments.

Experimenting with different carrier oils will help you discover which ones work best for your needs.

Chapter 4: Essential Oils Every Beginner Should Own

10 Essential Oils Every Beginner Should Own

When you first begin exploring the world of essential oils, the wide variety of options available can feel overwhelming. There are hundreds of essential oils extracted from plants around the world, each with its own unique aroma and potential benefits.

Fortunately, beginners do not need to purchase a large number of oils to get started. A small collection of versatile oils can provide a wide range of uses for physical wellness, emotional balance, and personal care.

The following ten essential oils are among the most popular and commonly recommended for beginners. These oils are widely used in aromatherapy and can easily become the foundation of your essential oil collection.

1. Lavender

Lavender essential oil is often considered the most versatile and beginner-friendly oil. It has a soft floral scent and is widely known for its calming properties.

Benefits

Lavender oil is commonly used to promote relaxation and emotional balance. Many people find that its soothing aroma helps reduce feelings of stress and tension. It is also frequently used in skincare routines because it may help support healthy-looking skin.

Lavender is especially popular for improving sleep quality. Its relaxing aroma can help prepare the mind and body for rest after a long day.

Common Uses

Lavender oil can be added to a diffuser in the evening to create a calming atmosphere before bedtime. Many people place a drop on their pillow or use it in a bedtime room spray.

It can also be diluted with a carrier oil and applied to the skin to soothe minor irritations or support relaxation during massage.

Safety Tips

Lavender is generally considered gentle when properly diluted. However, essential oils should always be diluted with a carrier oil before applying to the skin.

2. Tea Tree

Tea tree oil is well known for its powerful cleansing and purifying properties. It has a fresh, medicinal scent and is commonly used in natural skincare.

Benefits

Tea tree oil is widely used to help support clear skin because of its antibacterial and antifungal properties. It may also help maintain healthy nails and scalp.

Because of its cleansing qualities, tea tree oil is also used in many natural household cleaning products.

Common Uses

Tea tree oil is frequently added to skincare products designed for acne-prone skin. It can also be used in natural surface cleaners or added to shampoo to support scalp health.

Safety Tips

Tea tree oil should never be ingested. Always dilute it before applying it to the skin to reduce the risk of irritation.

3. Peppermint

Peppermint essential oil has a strong, refreshing aroma that is known for its energizing effects.

Benefits

Peppermint oil is often used to increase alertness and mental clarity. Many people also use it to help relieve tension headaches and soothe tired muscles.

Its cooling sensation makes it a popular ingredient in massage blends and topical treatments.

Common Uses

Peppermint oil can be diffused in a workspace to promote focus and concentration. When diluted with a carrier oil, it may be applied to the temples or neck to help relieve tension headaches.

It can also be used in massage blends to soothe sore muscles after exercise.

Safety Tips

Peppermint oil is very potent and should always be diluted before topical use. Avoid using peppermint oil on young children without professional guidance.

4. Lemon

Lemon essential oil has a bright, fresh citrus scent that many people find uplifting and energizing.

Benefits

Lemon oil is commonly used to boost mood and create a refreshing atmosphere. It also has cleansing properties that make it useful for natural cleaning products.

Many people enjoy using lemon oil to help promote mental clarity and a sense of freshness.

Common Uses

Lemon oil can be diffused in the home to create an uplifting environment. It is also frequently used in homemade cleaning sprays and air fresheners.

Safety Tips

Lemon oil can increase sensitivity to sunlight when applied to the skin. Avoid direct sun exposure for several hours after topical use.

5. Eucalyptus

Eucalyptus oil has a strong, crisp aroma often associated with respiratory support.

Benefits

Eucalyptus oil is commonly used to support clear breathing and relieve congestion. It may also help soothe tired muscles and create a refreshing atmosphere.

Its invigorating scent is frequently used in spa and wellness settings.

Common Uses

Eucalyptus oil is often used in steam inhalation to help clear nasal passages. It can also be added to massage oils to soothe sore muscles or diffused during cold and flu season.

Safety Tips

Avoid using eucalyptus oil on young children unless recommended by a healthcare professional. Always dilute before applying to the skin.

6. Frankincense

Frankincense has been used for thousands of years in traditional practices and spiritual rituals. It has a warm, woody aroma that many people find grounding.

Benefits

Frankincense oil is often used to promote relaxation and emotional balance. It is also popular in skincare routines because it may help support healthy-looking skin.

Many people use frankincense during meditation or relaxation practices.

Common Uses

Frankincense can be diffused to create a calming environment. It is also commonly added to facial oils or creams for skincare routines.

Safety Tips

Frankincense is generally considered safe when properly diluted. As with all essential oils, perform a small patch test before applying it to the skin.

7. Rosemary

Rosemary essential oil has a stimulating herbal aroma that

is known for promoting focus and mental clarity.

Benefits

Rosemary oil is often used to improve concentration and memory. It is also widely used in hair care products because it may support healthy hair growth.

Common Uses

Many people add rosemary oil to shampoos or scalp treatments. It can also be diffused in a workspace to help maintain focus during studying or working.

Safety Tips

People with certain medical conditions, including high blood pressure, should consult a healthcare professional before using rosemary oil.

8. Chamomile

Chamomile essential oil is known for its gentle, soothing properties.

Benefits

Chamomile oil is often used to promote relaxation and reduce feelings of stress. It may also help soothe irritated or sensitive skin.

Common Uses

Chamomile oil can be added to a bath or diffuser to

encourage relaxation before sleep. It is also commonly used in skincare blends designed for sensitive skin.

Safety Tips

Individuals who are allergic to ragweed or similar plants should use chamomile oil with caution.

9. Orange

Sweet orange essential oil has a bright, cheerful citrus aroma that many people find uplifting.

Benefits

Orange oil is often used to boost mood and reduce feelings of stress. Its refreshing scent can help create a warm and welcoming atmosphere in the home.

Common Uses

Orange oil is commonly used in diffusers, room sprays, and natural cleaning products. It can also be blended with other citrus oils to create uplifting aromas.

Safety Tips

Like many citrus oils, orange oil can increase skin sensitivity to sunlight when applied topically.

10. Clary Sage

Clary sage essential oil has a warm, herbaceous scent that is often associated with relaxation and emotional balance.

Benefits

Clary sage is commonly used to promote relaxation and help ease emotional tension. It is also widely used in aromatherapy blends designed to support hormonal balance.

Common Uses

Clary sage oil can be used in massage oils, bath blends, or diffusers to promote relaxation and emotional comfort.

Safety Tips

Clary sage should be avoided during pregnancy unless recommended by a qualified healthcare professional.

Chapter 5: Everyday Aromatherapy

20 Diffuser Blends for Everyday Life

One of the easiest and most enjoyable ways to use essential oils is with a diffuser. Diffusers disperse tiny particles of essential oils into the air, allowing you to experience their aroma throughout a room.

Diffusing essential oils can help create a relaxing atmosphere, improve focus, uplift mood, or simply make your home smell pleasant and refreshing.

The following blends are simple combinations that beginners can easily prepare using common essential oils. Add the recommended number of drops to your diffuser filled with water according to the manufacturer's instructions.

Relaxation and Stress Relief

1. Calm Evening Blend

- 3 drops Lavender
- 2 drops Frankincense
- 2 drops Orange

This blend helps create a peaceful environment after a long day and supports relaxation.

2. Stress Relief Blend

- 3 drops Lavender
- 2 drops Bergamot
- 1 drop Chamomile

This blend may help calm the mind and reduce feelings of tension.

3. Meditation Blend

- 3 drops Frankincense
- 2 drops Sandalwood
- 1 drop Lavender

Ideal for meditation, yoga, or quiet reflection.

Sleep and Rest

4. Deep Sleep Blend

- 4 drops Lavender
- 2 drops Chamomile
- 1 drop Clary Sage

Diffuse this blend in the evening to help create a restful atmosphere before bedtime.

5. Bedtime Calm Blend

- 3 drops Lavender
- 2 drops Cedarwood
- 1 drop Orange

This gentle blend supports relaxation and prepares the mind for sleep.

Energy and Focus

6. Morning Energy Blend

- 3 drops Lemon
- 2 drops Peppermint
- 1 drop Rosemary

This refreshing blend is perfect for starting the day with clarity and energy.

7. Focus Blend

- 3 drops Rosemary
- 2 drops Lemon
- 1 drop Peppermint

Ideal for studying, reading, or working.

8. Mental Clarity Blend

- 2 drops Peppermint

- 2 drops Lemon
- 2 drops Eucalyptus

Helps promote alertness and mental focus.

Mood Boosting Blends

9. Happy Mood Blend

- 3 drops Orange
- 2 drops Lemon
- 1 drop Bergamot

This uplifting citrus blend may help improve mood.

10. Positive Energy Blend

- 3 drops Grapefruit
- 2 drops Lemon
- 1 drop Peppermint

A bright and refreshing aroma that helps energize the room.

11. Cheerful Home Blend

- 3 drops Orange
- 2 drops Lavender
- 1 drop Lemon

Creates a warm and welcoming environment.

Respiratory Support

12. Clear Breathing Blend

- 3 drops Eucalyptus
- 2 drops Peppermint
- 1 drop Tea Tree

Often used during cold and flu season to help clear the airways.

13. Fresh Air Blend

- 3 drops Lemon
- 2 drops Eucalyptus
- 1 drop Tea Tree

Helps refresh and purify the air in your home.

Relaxing Home Atmosphere

14. Spa Blend

- 3 drops Lavender
- 2 drops Eucalyptus
- 1 drop Peppermint

Creates a spa-like atmosphere at home.

15. Peaceful Home Blend

- 3 drops Frankincense
- 2 drops Orange
- 1 drop Lavender

A calming blend for relaxation and quiet evenings.

Seasonal Blends

16. Autumn Comfort Blend

- 3 drops Orange
- 2 drops Clove
- 1 drop Cinnamon

Creates a warm and cozy atmosphere during cooler months.

17. Winter Fresh Blend

- 3 drops Pine
- 2 drops Eucalyptus
- 1 drop Peppermint

A refreshing blend often used during winter.

Clean and Refreshing Blends

18. Fresh Home Blend

- 3 drops Lemon
- 2 drops Tea Tree

- 1 drop Eucalyptus

Helps freshen the air and eliminate odors.

19. Kitchen Fresh Blend

- 3 drops Lemon
- 2 drops Orange
- 1 drop Peppermint

Great for removing cooking odors.

Uplifting Blend

20. Sunshine Blend

- 3 drops Orange
- 2 drops Grapefruit
- 1 drop Lemon

A bright citrus blend that creates an uplifting atmosphere.

Tips for Using Diffuser Blends

- Always follow the instructions provided with your diffuser.
- Start with fewer drops and increase if necessary.
- Diffuse essential oils for 30–60 minutes at a time.
- Make sure the room is well ventilated.
- Avoid diffusing oils continuously for long periods.

Using diffuser blends is one of the simplest ways to

experience the benefits of aromatherapy. With just a few essential oils, you can create a variety of aromas that support relaxation, focus, and overall well-being.

Chapter 6: Essential Oils For Health

Essential Oils For Health

Essential oils have been used for centuries in traditional practices to support physical well-being. Today, many people use them as part of their wellness routines to help promote relaxation, ease minor discomforts, and support overall health.

It is important to remember that aromatherapy is considered a complementary practice. Essential oils should not replace professional medical care. If you are dealing with a serious health condition or taking medication, it is always best to consult a healthcare professional before using essential oils.

Below are some of the most commonly used essential oils that may help support health and wellness.

1. Clove

Clove essential oil is known for its strong, warm aroma and

powerful antibacterial properties.

Benefits

Clove oil may help support the immune system and provide relief for minor discomforts. It has traditionally been used for toothaches and infections because of its antiseptic properties.

Common Uses

Clove oil is sometimes used in diluted form for oral care or massage blends designed to soothe sore muscles and joints. It may also be diffused during cold and flu season to help purify the air.

Safety Tips

Clove oil is very potent and should always be diluted with a carrier oil before applying to the skin.

2. Cypress

Cypress essential oil has a fresh, clean aroma and is often associated with circulation and respiratory support.

Benefits

Cypress oil may help support healthy circulation and muscle relaxation. It is sometimes used to help relieve muscle cramps and support respiratory comfort.

Common Uses

It can be used in massage oils for tired legs or muscles. Many people also diffuse cypress oil to promote a calming and refreshing atmosphere.

Safety Tips

Always dilute cypress oil before applying it to the skin.

3. Eucalyptus

Eucalyptus oil is widely known for its refreshing scent and respiratory benefits.

Benefits

Eucalyptus oil is often used to help support clear breathing and relieve congestion. It may also help soothe sore muscles.

Common Uses

Many people add eucalyptus oil to steam inhalations or diffusers during cold and flu season. It is also used in massage oils for muscle discomfort.

Safety Tips

Avoid using eucalyptus oil on young children without professional advice.

4. Frankincense

Frankincense essential oil has a warm, woody aroma that has been valued for centuries.

Benefits

Frankincense oil is often used to promote relaxation and emotional balance. It may also support healthy skin and overall wellness.

Common Uses

Frankincense is commonly used in diffusers during meditation or relaxation practices. It is also popular in skincare blends.

Safety Tips

Perform a patch test before applying frankincense oil to the skin.

5. Ginger

Ginger essential oil has a warm and spicy scent.

Benefits

Ginger oil may help support digestion and relieve minor stomach discomfort. It is also commonly used to soothe sore muscles and improve circulation.

Common Uses

It can be used in massage blends for muscle discomfort or diffused to create a warm and energizing atmosphere.

Safety Tips

Always dilute ginger oil before applying to the skin, as it can be strong and warming.

6. Lavender

Lavender essential oil is one of the most widely used oils in aromatherapy.

Benefits

Lavender oil is known for its calming properties and may help promote relaxation and better sleep. It is also used to soothe minor skin irritations.

Common Uses

Lavender oil can be diffused before bedtime to promote restful sleep. It may also be diluted and applied to the skin for relaxation or minor skin care.

Safety Tips

Lavender is generally gentle, but it should still be diluted before topical use.

7. Myrrh

Myrrh essential oil has been used in traditional medicine for centuries.

Benefits

Myrrh oil may support skin health and promote relaxation.

It has also been used historically to help soothe wounds and inflammation.

Common Uses

It is often added to skincare products or diffused to create a calming atmosphere.

Safety Tips

Always dilute myrrh oil before applying to the skin.

8. Orange

Sweet orange essential oil has a bright citrus scent that many people find uplifting.

Benefits

Orange oil may help improve mood and reduce feelings of stress. It can also help freshen indoor air.

Common Uses

It is commonly used in diffusers, room sprays, and natural cleaning products.

Safety Tips

Orange oil can increase sensitivity to sunlight when applied to the skin.

9. Peppermint

Peppermint oil is known for its cooling sensation and refreshing aroma.

Benefits

Peppermint oil may help relieve headaches, improve focus, and soothe muscle discomfort.

Common Uses

It can be diffused to promote alertness or diluted and applied to the temples for tension headaches.

Safety Tips

Peppermint oil is very strong and should always be diluted before use.

10. Sandalwood

Sandalwood essential oil has a warm, woody aroma that promotes relaxation.

Benefits

Sandalwood oil may help promote calmness and emotional balance. It is also used in skincare products.

Common Uses

It can be diffused during meditation or relaxation practices.

Safety Tips

Always dilute sandalwood oil before applying it to the skin.

Essential Oils Recipes For Health Problems

When using essential oils on your skin, it is best to dilute them in a carrier. A carrier can be an organic oil for example. The best organic oil to use is jojoba. It is crucial to know how much essential oil you should put in the carrier. The dilution ratio of 1%, 2% or 3%.

For example:

1% dilution for 30 ml, add 5 to 6 drops.
2% dilution for 30 ml, add 10 to 12 drops and
3% dilution for 30 ml, add 15 to 18 drops.

I would like to give some recipes on the seven common everyday heath problems and how to deal with them with essential oils.

1) Bloating

Some reasons why people suffer from bloating is that they overeat, or have an excess of gas or because of certain foods like cabbage, cauliflower, etc

Ingredients

3 drops of peppermint (antifungal, anti-inflammatory,

stimulating to the circulatory system, and analgesic, used to aid digestion)
4 drops of ginger (help bring balance to the digestive system.)
30 ml of jojoba oil

Instructions:

Blend the lotion and the oils.
Massage some of the lotion onto the area of discomfort and some onto the point located on the side of the inner side of the foot, four finger widths away from the big toe. This is the acupressure point that relieves indigestion, stomach ache, and nausea.

2) Constipation

Some reasons of constipation are poor diet, hormonal imbalance, lack of activity, stress and not drinking enough water

Ingredients

3 drops Mandarin (antiseptic, antispasmodic, diuretic and is a laxative and digestive)
3 drops Rosemary (enhances digestive system circulation to boost the elimination of waste products)
3 drops Ginger (eases inflammation and digestive problems, helps to relax the intestines and improve gastric motility)
30 ml of jojoba oil

Instructions:
Blend all the oils and massage over the abdomen and

lower back daily for 6 to 8 weeks.
It is better to do it once a week after the evening bath.

3) PMS

PMS, known as premenstrual syndrome, is related to the fluctuating levels of hormones, including estrogens and progesterone, that occur in preparation for menstruation
Ingredients

2 drops Chamomile (antispasmodic, antidepressant, anti-inflammatory)
5 drops anise (eases menstrual pain)
8 drops clary sage (helps to reduce stress, alleviate pain and balance hormones.
30 ml grapeseed carrier oil

Instructions:
Apply this blend to the abdomen, every night and morning immediately after finishing menstruating each month till the next period commences.

Also, twice a week, use this blend in the bath. Keep the treatment for about six months.
Then stop the morning application and keep making the application only at night for two months

4) Sinus

According to Medicine Net, sinus infection is the inflammation of the air cavities within the passages of the nose. Allergies and chemicals can cause it

Ingredients

3 drops of pine (reduce inflammation, protect against sinus infections, clear mucus, and phlegm
3 drops of eucalyptus (eliminate inflammation, boost respiratory health)
3 drops of peppermint (respiratory problems and pain)
1 tsp of sesame oil

Instructions:
Blend the essential oils together with the sesame oil.
Massage into your face around the eyes and onto the cheekbones and also your eyebrows and forehead to relieve the sinus pressure.

Do not get near the eyes.

5) Muscle pain

Ingredients

7 drops cedar wood (antispasmodic, tonic, sedative and anti-inflammatory)
3 drops peppermint (anti-inflammatory, antispasmodic and relieves pain)
7 drops Ravensara (antispasmodic, analgesic, disinfectant, smooth muscle pain)
30 ml of jojoba oil

Instructions:
Blend the essential oils with the jojoba oil. Rub a little of the blend on your wrists, along the sides of your neck or on your chest.
Try the sore muscle blend on a tense or painful muscle or joint.
Apply before bedtime.

6) Insomnia

Insomnia is the inability to sleep or the inability to go back to sleep once one wakes up in the middle of the night. Research has found that while sleeping the body regulates hormones and recharges the immune system. This is why is so important to have a good night sleep to preserve your health. Some causes of insomnia are stress, anxiety, depression, etc

Ingredients

8 drops Lavender (relaxation and sedative)
8 drops Chamomile (sedative and relaxing properties)
8 drops Sweet Marjoram (calming, sedative, helps ease nervous tension, soothe grief, loneliness, and rejection)
8 oz. distilled water
A spray container

Instructions:
Mix the essential oils and put them into the spray container, shake well and spray around the bedroom and onto your pillow.

7) Headaches

There are several causes of a headache. One of the most common causes is headache caused by digestive disorders. In that case, the best essential oil is peppermint.

3 drops peppermint

Directions:
Drop the 3 drops of peppermint onto your fingers and massage your forehead and temples. Avoid putting the oil near your eyes.

8) Cold Relief

Colds are common infections that may cause congestion, fatigue, and coughing. Essential oils may help support breathing comfort and relaxation.

Ingredients

3 drops eucalyptus
2 drops peppermint
2 drops tea tree
1 tablespoon carrier oil

Instructions
Blend the essential oils with the carrier oil.
Massage gently onto the chest and upper back.
You can also diffuse this blend in a room to help create a refreshing environment.

9) Cough Relief

Coughing may occur due to colds, irritation of the throat, or respiratory infections.

Ingredients

3 drops of eucalyptus
2 drops lavender
2 drops of lemon

1 tablespoon carrier oil

Instructions
Mix the oils with the carrier oil.
Massage lightly onto the chest and throat area.

10) Digestive Support

Digestive discomfort may occur after heavy meals or poor digestion.

Ingredients

3 drops of ginger
2 drops peppermint
1 tablespoon jojoba oil

Instructions
Blend the oils with the carrier oil and massage gently onto the abdomen using circular motions.

11) Stress Relief

Stress is a common issue in modern life and can affect both physical and emotional health.

Ingredients

3 drops lavender
2 drops frankincense
2 drops of orange
1 tablespoon carrier oil

Instructions

Blend the oils with the carrier oil and massage onto the neck and shoulders.

12) Anxiety Relief

Feelings of anxiety can sometimes cause tension, restlessness, or difficulty concentrating.

Ingredients

3 drops lavender
2 drops bergamot
1 drop chamomile
1 tablespoon carrier oil

Instructions

Massage onto the wrists and inhale the aroma deeply.

13) Fatigue

Fatigue may occur due to lack of sleep, stress, or physical exhaustion.

Ingredients

3 drops peppermint
2 drops lemon
2 drops rosemary
1 tablespoon carrier oil

Instructions
Massage onto the neck and shoulders or diffuse in the

room to help promote alertness.

14) Immune Support

Supporting the immune system can help the body remain strong and resilient.

Ingredients

3 drops lemon
2 drops tea tree
2 drops eucalyptus
1 tablespoon carrier oil

Instructions
Massage onto the chest or diffuse in the home during cold and flu season.

15) Joint Pain

Joint discomfort may occur due to physical activity or aging.

Ingredients

4 drops ginger
3 drops peppermint
1 tablespoon carrier oil

Instructions

Massage gently onto the affected joints.

16) Nausea

Nausea may occur during travel, digestive upset, or illness.

Ingredients

3 drops ginger
2 drops peppermint
1 tablespoon carrier oil
Instructions
Massage lightly onto the abdomen or inhale the aroma from your palms.

17) Poor Circulation

Poor circulation can cause cold hands and feet or muscle fatigue.

Ingredients

3 drops rosemary
2 drops ginger
1 tablespoon carrier oil

Instructions
Massage onto the legs and feet to help stimulate circulation.

Recipe Disclaimer

The recipes in this book are provided for educational and informational purposes only. Essential oils are highly concentrated and should always be used responsibly and properly diluted before topical use. If you have a medical condition, are pregnant, or are taking medication, consult a qualified healthcare professional before using essential oils.

Chapter 7: Essential Oils For Emotional Well-Being

Essential Oils For Negative Emotions

Anger : Lavender, lemon,ylang-ylang, roman chamomile, wild orange
Anxiety : Cedarwood,Bergamot,sandalwood
Stress :   Bergamot, lavender,lemon,peppermint
Fear : Cedarwood, ginger,sandalwood
Grief : Bergamot, Roman chamomile, eucalyptus,lavender

Recipes For Negative Emotions

For negative emotions in my opinion, I think is better to use only one essential oil rather than a recipe. Emotions come out suddenly, and we need a quick and fast solution. It is easier to add 1 or 2 drops of essential oil for that particular emotion in a tissue and breathe deeply than to make a recipe.

We can even carry the essential oil bottle with us, and if something comes up at the job, for example, we just pull the bottle, add the drops to a tissue, and we will feel better in minutes. The most common negative emotions we feel every day are:

1) Anger

One of the best essential oils to control anger is Rose oil. According to Dr. Oz, this oil can be used to calm anger, lighten feelings of resentment, jealousy, and grief.
According to Ayurveda, the rose has three main medicinal properties:

It is smoothing, moisturizing and cooling. Rose oil on its own is considered a powerful tool against anger and other emotional wounds, instilling compassion and forgiveness.
Add 1-2 drops to a tissue and breathe in deeply all through the day for an anger management solution on the go.

2) Sadness

Among the best essential oils for sadness are lemon, lime, grapefruit, orange, and peppermint. These essential oils help to make you feel happy.
Add 1 – 2 drops to a tissue and breathe in deeply. You can also take a warm bath. Add to the bath tab 5 to 10 drops of any of these oils and relax.

3) Jealousy

Often when we feel jealousy can cause a tightening of the chest, a shortness of breath, and a shallow airy breathing pattern. Because this emotion affects our heart the essential oils that might help are eucalyptus, peppermint, rosemary, rose, chamomile, marjoram, sandalwood, and

frankincense.
Add 1-2 drops of any of the essential oils mentioned before to a tissue and breathe deeply.

4) Worthlessness

A pilot study involving 24 professionals from a nursing group was carried in Portugal to verify the use of ylang-ylang essential oil in relieving anxiety and increasing self-esteem. The results showed clear evidence that the use of ylang-ylang led to a significant alteration in self-esteem.
Add 3 drops of ylang-ylang to a tissue and breathe in deeply twice a day.

5) Anxiety

Depending on the situation or intention, many other essential oils may be appropriate. For example, a person experiencing lots of anxiety that manifests in excessive worry, overthinking and sleeplessness will likely be restless and ungrounded.
Such a person may benefit from Bay Laurel, Clary Sage or Cypress, which addresses the underlying emotions.

Chapter 8: Essential Oils For Beauty

Essential Oils For Beauty

Essential oils are used for body care, face, and hair. You can find a lot of skin products for body care, face and hair, but you can also make your own. Some essential oils for skin and hair care are:

Rose: Helps balance moisture levels in the skin and reduces the appearance of skin imperfections.
Rosemary: Used in hair care in shampoos and lotions because it stimulates follicles, thus making the hair grow longer and stronger. It is also known to slow down premature hair loss.

Lavender is analgesic, antibacterial, and antiseptic, and it is used for acne. Ylan is also good for acne because it has antimicrobial and astringent properties.
Frankincense has anti-inflammatory and anti-microbial properties. It is used for treating aging skin because it tightens and firms, and it minimizes age spots and dark marks.

Essential Oils Recipes For Beauty

Most common beauty concerns are skin and hair care.

Acne

Ingredients

6 drops lavender (analgesic, antibacterial, and antiseptic)
5 drops tea tree (antibacterial, cicatrizing, antimicrobial, antiseptic, antiviral,fungicide)
1 drop geranium (astringent,cicatrizant, tonic, reduce inflammation and irritation)
30 ml jojoba oil

Instructions:
Mix the ingredients and apply a small amount to the face once a day, avoid eyes and lips.

Anti-aging

Ingredients

3 drops frankincense (anti-inflammatory and anti-microbial property. It is used for treating aging skin because it tightens and firm, minimize age spots and dark marks)
3 drops Rose (improve circulation and help maintain the elasticity of the skin)
3 drops cypress (improves circulation, antibacterial, anti-infectious and anti-microbial, is a firming oil)
30 ml sweet almond oil (contains vitamin E that helps to fight wrinkles and firms the skin)

Instructions:
Mix the essential oils with the sweet almond oil.
Use it in the morning and at night.
Spread on your face, avoid the eyes.

Hair grow

Ingredients:

8 drops rosemary
5 ml jojoba oil

Instructions:
Mix the rosemary oil with the jojoba oil.
Put some of the mixture on your fingertips and massage into your scalp.
You can apply it in the morning and before going to bed

Dry Skin Moisturizing Oil

Dry skin can become rough, itchy, and irritated. Essential oils blended with nourishing carrier oils can help support skin hydration.

Ingredients

4 drops lavender
3 drops geranium
2 drops frankincense
30 ml sweet almond oil

Instructions

Mix the essential oils with the carrier oil.
Apply a small amount to dry areas of the skin once or twice daily.

Natural Facial Cleanser

This gentle blend can help cleanse the skin and maintain a healthy appearance.

Ingredients

3 drops tea tree
2 drops lavender
1 tablespoon jojoba oil

Instructions
Mix the oils together and massage gently onto the face.
Rinse with warm water and pat dry.

Face Serum for Glowing Skin

Essential oils can help support healthy and radiant skin.

Ingredients

3 drops frankincense
2 drops lavender
1 drop geranium
30 ml jojoba oil

Instructions
Blend the oils and apply a few drops to the face at night before going to bed.

Dandruff Treatment

Dandruff may occur when the scalp becomes dry or irritated.

Ingredients

4 drops tea tree
3 drops rosemary
1 tablespoon coconut oil

Instructions
Massage the blend into the scalp and leave it on for 20–30 minutes before washing the hair.

Natural Lip Care Oil

This blend may help soothe dry or cracked lips.

Ingredients

2 drops lavender
1 tablespoon coconut oil

Instructions
Mix the oils together and apply a small amount to the lips when needed.

Stretch Mark Oil

Stretch marks may appear after weight changes or pregnancy.

Ingredients

3 drops lavender
2 drops frankincense
30 ml rosehip oil

Instructions
Massage gently onto the affected area once or twice daily.

Relaxing Bath Oil

A relaxing bath can help reduce stress and improve well-being.

Ingredients

4 drops lavender
3 drops chamomile
1 tablespoon carrier oil

Instructions
Add the mixture to warm bath water and soak for 15–20 minutes.

Chapter 9: DIY Essential Oil Home Products

Essential oils are not only useful for personal care and wellness, but they can also be used to create simple and natural products for your home. Many commercial products contain synthetic fragrances and chemicals, while homemade alternatives allow you to control the ingredients and enjoy natural aromas.

The following recipes are easy to prepare and require only a few ingredients.

Natural Cleaning Spray

This simple cleaning spray can help clean surfaces while leaving a fresh scent.

Ingredients

10 drops lemon essential oil
10 drops tea tree essential oil
1 cup distilled water
½ cup white vinegar

Instructions

Pour the water and vinegar into a spray bottle.
Add the essential oils and shake well before each use.

How to Use

Spray onto kitchen counters, sinks, and other surfaces, then wipe with a clean cloth.

Linen Spray

A linen spray can help freshen pillows, bedding, and curtains.

Ingredients

8 drops lavender essential oil
5 drops chamomile essential oil
1 cup distilled water

Instructions

Add the essential oils to a spray bottle filled with distilled water. Shake well before each use.

How to Use

Lightly spray onto pillows, sheets, or curtains to create a relaxing aroma.

Natural Air Freshener

This blend can help remove odors and create a pleasant atmosphere in your home.

Ingredients

6 drops orange essential oil
4 drops lemon essential oil

2 drops lavender essential oil
1 cup distilled water

Instructions

Combine the ingredients in a spray bottle and shake well before spraying.

How to Use

Spray into the air in any room to refresh the environment.

Natural Perfume

Essential oils can be used to create a simple natural fragrance.

Ingredients

5 drops lavender
3 drops orange
2 drops frankincense
10 ml jojoba oil

Instructions

Mix the oils in a small glass bottle and shake gently.

How to Use

Apply a small amount to the wrists or behind the ears.

Relaxing Bath Salts

Bath salts can help create a soothing and relaxing bath experience.

Ingredients

1 cup Epsom salt
5 drops lavender essential oil
3 drops of chamomile essential oil

Instructions

Mix the ingredients in a bowl and store in a sealed container.

How to Use

Add a handful of the bath salts to warm bath water and relax for 15–20 minutes.

Massage Oil

Massage oils can help relax muscles and relieve tension.

Ingredients

5 drops lavender
3 drops peppermint
30 ml sweet almond oil

Instructions

Mix the oils together in a small bottle.

How to Use

Massage gently into the shoulders, neck, or back.

Natural Bathroom Cleaner

Essential oils can also be used to help clean bathroom surfaces.

Ingredients

10 drops tea tree oil
10 drops lemon oil
1 cup water
½ cup vinegar

Instructions

Combine all ingredients in a spray bottle and shake before use.

How to Use

Spray onto sinks, tiles, and other bathroom surfaces and wipe clean.

Natural Carpet Freshener

This blend can help freshen carpets and eliminate odors.

Ingredients

1 cup baking soda
10 drops lavender essential oil
5 drops lemon essential oil

Instructions

Mix the baking soda and oils in a bowl.

How to Use

Sprinkle lightly over the carpet, leave for 15 minutes, then vacuum.

Closet Freshener

A natural way to keep closets smelling fresh.

Ingredients

3 drops lavender
3 drops lemon
Cotton balls

Instructions

Place the drops of essential oils on cotton balls and place them in small containers inside the closet.

Natural Hand Massage Oil

This simple blend helps soften and moisturize the hands.

Ingredients

3 drops lavender
2 drops geranium
1 tablespoon sweet almond oil

Instructions

Blend the oils together and massage gently into the hands.

Chapter 10: Essential Oil Safety Guide

Essential oils are powerful plant extracts that should always be used with care. While they offer many potential benefits, improper use may cause irritation or other unwanted reactions.

Understanding the basic safety guidelines will help ensure that essential oils are used safely and effectively.

Dilution Guidelines

Essential oils are highly concentrated and should usually be diluted before applying them to the skin. Carrier oils help dilute essential oils and make them safer for topical use.

Common carrier oils include:

Jojoba oil

Sweet almond oil

Coconut oil

Grapeseed oil

Olive oil

General Dilution Guidelines

1% dilution
5–6 drops of essential oil per 30 ml of carrier oil
Recommended for sensitive skin, elderly people, and children.

2% dilution
10–12 drops of essential oil per 30 ml of carrier oil
Suitable for everyday use.

3% dilution
15–18 drops of essential oil per 30 ml of carrier oil
Often used for short-term treatments.

Perform a Patch Test

Before applying any new essential oil to the skin, it is recommended to perform a patch test.

Apply a small diluted amount of the oil to a small area of skin, such as the inside of the wrist or elbow. Wait 24 hours to see if any irritation occurs.

If redness, itching, or irritation appears, discontinue use.

Avoid Contact With Eyes and Sensitive Areas

Essential oils should never be applied directly to the eyes, inside the ears, or other sensitive areas of the body.

If essential oil accidentally comes into contact with the eyes, do not rinse with water. Instead, apply a carrier oil to help dilute the essential oil and reduce irritation.

Use Caution During Pregnancy

Some essential oils should be avoided during pregnancy. Always consult a qualified healthcare professional before using essential oils during pregnancy.

Children and Essential Oils

Children have more sensitive skin than adults. Essential oils should always be diluted more carefully when used for children.

Some oils, such as peppermint and eucalyptus, should be used with caution around young children.

Pets and Essential Oils

Pets may be sensitive to certain essential oils. Avoid diffusing essential oils in enclosed spaces where pets cannot leave the area.

If you plan to use essential oils around pets, consult a veterinarian for guidance.

Storage of Essential Oils

To preserve their quality and safety, essential oils should be stored properly.

Keep essential oils:

In dark glass bottles

Away from direct sunlight

In a cool, dry place

Out of reach of children and pets

Proper storage helps maintain the quality and effectiveness of essential oils.

Use Essential Oils Responsibly

Essential oils can be a valuable addition to a healthy lifestyle when used responsibly. By following proper safety guidelines, you can enjoy their aromas and benefits while minimizing potential risks.

Always remember that aromatherapy should complement, not replace, professional medical care.

Chapter 11: How to Start Your Essential Oil Collection

Beginning your essential oil journey can feel overwhelming at first. With so many different oils available, many beginners are unsure where to start or which oils they should purchase first.

Fortunately, you do not need a large collection to begin enjoying the benefits of aromatherapy. Starting with a small selection of versatile oils will allow you to experiment with different blends and uses while learning how essential oils work.

With a few carefully chosen oils and some basic tools, you can begin creating your own natural remedies, diffuser blends, and personal care products.

Choosing Your First Essential Oils

When starting your collection, it is best to begin with oils that have many uses. These oils can be used for relaxation, skincare, respiratory support, and everyday wellness.
Some of the most popular beginner oils include:

Lavender – known for relaxation and sleep support
Peppermint – commonly used for headaches and mental clarity

Lemon – uplifting and refreshing, often used in cleaning products
Tea Tree – popular for skin care and natural cleansing
Eucalyptus – commonly used for respiratory support
Frankincense – valued for relaxation and skincare

These oils provide a strong foundation and can be combined to create many different blends.

Understanding Essential Oil Quality

Not all essential oils are created equal. High-quality oils are typically produced through careful distillation or cold pressing of plant materials.

When choosing essential oils, look for products that clearly state the botanical name of the plant, the country of origin, and the method of extraction.

Pure essential oils should not contain synthetic fragrances or additives. Choosing high-quality oils ensures better aroma and safer use.

Basic Tools You Will Need

In addition to essential oils, a few simple tools can help you use them safely and effectively.

Diffuser
A diffuser disperses essential oils into the air, allowing you to enjoy their aroma throughout a room. Diffusers are one of the easiest ways to experience aromatherapy.

Carrier Oils

Carrier oils are used to dilute essential oils before applying them to the skin. Common carrier oils include:

Jojoba oil
Sweet almond oil
Coconut oil
Grapeseed oil

Small Glass Bottles

Glass bottles are useful for storing blends and homemade products. Dark glass bottles help protect essential oils from sunlight.

Droppers and Measuring Tools

These help ensure accurate dilution when preparing blends.

Storing Your Essential Oils

Proper storage helps preserve the quality and effectiveness of essential oils.
To protect your oils:

- Store them in dark glass bottles
- Keep them away from heat and sunlight
- Store them in a cool, dry place
- Keep them out of reach of children and pets

When stored properly, many essential oils can maintain their quality for several years.

Building Your Collection Over Time

As you become more comfortable using essential oils, you may want to expand your collection.
You might consider adding oils such as:

Rosemary – often used for hair and mental focus
Chamomile – known for calming properties
Geranium – popular in skincare blends
Orange – uplifting citrus aroma
Clary Sage – commonly used for relaxation

There is no need to rush when building your collection. Over time you will discover which oils you enjoy most and which ones work best for your needs.

Tips for Beginners

If you are new to essential oils, the following tips may help you get started safely.

• Start with a small number of oils
• Always dilute oils before applying them to the skin
• Perform a patch test before using a new oil
• Follow recommended dilution guidelines
• Learn about each oil before using it

With practice and knowledge, essential oils can become a valuable part of your daily wellness routine.

Chapter 12: Essential Oils Quick Reference Guide

This quick reference guide provides an overview of commonly used essential oils and their most popular applications. It is designed to help you quickly identify which oils may be useful for different situations.

While this guide offers helpful suggestions, always remember to use essential oils safely and consult a healthcare professional if you have a medical condition.

Essential Oils for Relaxation and Stress

Lavender

Lavender is one of the most widely used oils for relaxation and emotional balance. Its gentle floral aroma can help calm the mind and reduce feelings of stress.

Common uses include diffusing before bedtime, adding to bath blends, or using in massage oils.

Chamomile

Chamomile oil is known for its soothing and calming properties. It is often used to help promote restful sleep and relaxation.

It can be diffused in the evening or added to bath water.

Clary Sage

Clary sage has a warm herbal aroma that helps promote emotional balance. It is commonly used to help reduce stress and tension.

Frankincense
Frankincense has been valued for centuries for its grounding aroma. It is often used during meditation and relaxation practices.

Essential Oils for Energy and Focus

Peppermint
Peppermint oil has a refreshing aroma that helps increase alertness and mental clarity. It is often used when studying or working.

Lemon
Lemon oil has a bright citrus scent that can uplift mood and promote concentration.

Rosemary
Rosemary oil is commonly used to improve focus, concentration, and memory.

Eucalyptus
Eucalyptus oil has a refreshing scent that may help increase mental alertness.

Essential Oils for Skin Care

Tea Tree
Tea tree oil is well known for its cleansing and antibacterial

properties. It is often used to support clear skin.

Lavender
Lavender oil may help soothe irritated skin and promote skin healing.

Frankincense
Frankincense is widely used in anti-aging skincare blends and may help support healthy-looking skin.

Geranium
Geranium oil helps balance the skin's natural oils and is often used in facial care blends.

Essential Oils for Respiratory Support

Eucalyptus
Eucalyptus oil is often used to support clear breathing and relieve congestion.

Peppermint
Peppermint oil provides a cooling sensation and may help ease respiratory discomfort.

Tea Tree
Tea tree oil is commonly used in diffusers during cold and flu season.

Pine
Pine oil has a fresh aroma that may help support respiratory comfort.

Essential Oils for Digestive Support

Ginger
Ginger oil may help support digestion and reduce stomach discomfort.

Peppermint
Peppermint oil is often used to help relieve bloating and indigestion.

Orange
Orange oil may help stimulate digestion and improve mood.

Essential Oils for Emotional Balance

Rose
Rose oil has traditionally been used to support emotional well-being and calm feelings of sadness.

Ylang-Ylang
Ylang-ylang is often used to promote relaxation and emotional comfort.

Bergamot
Bergamot oil has an uplifting aroma and is commonly used to support a positive mood.

Essential Oils for Pain Relief

Peppermint
Peppermint oil is often used to help relieve headaches and

muscle discomfort.

Ginger
Ginger oil may help soothe sore muscles and joints.

Lavender
Lavender oil is frequently used in massage blends to relax muscles.

Eucalyptus
Eucalyptus oil is commonly used to help soothe tired muscles.

Essential Oils for Sleep

Lavender
Lavender is widely used to promote restful sleep and relaxation.

Chamomile
Chamomile oil helps calm the mind and prepare the body for sleep.

Clary Sage
Clary sage can help create a relaxing nighttime environment.

Quick Safety Reminder

Always dilute essential oils before applying them to the skin. Some oils may cause skin irritation or sensitivity to sunlight. When in doubt, perform a patch test before using a new oil.

Essential oils should be used as a complementary wellness practice and should not replace professional medical care.

Frequently Asked Questions

What Are Essential Oils?

Essential oils are concentrated extracts obtained from plants such as flowers, leaves, bark, roots, and fruits. These oils capture the plant's natural aroma and many of its beneficial properties. They are commonly used in aromatherapy to support relaxation, emotional balance, and general well-being.

Because essential oils are highly concentrated, only a small amount is needed to experience their aroma and potential benefits.

Can Essential Oils Be Applied Directly to the Skin?

Most essential oils should not be applied directly to the skin without dilution. Because they are highly concentrated, undiluted oils may cause skin irritation or sensitivity.

For topical use, essential oils should be diluted with a carrier oil such as jojoba oil, sweet almond oil, coconut oil, or grapeseed oil. Carrier oils help reduce the strength of essential oils and allow them to be safely absorbed by the skin.

Always perform a patch test before applying a new oil to a larger area of the body.

What Is the Best Way to Use Essential Oils?

There are several ways to use essential oils depending on your needs.
The most common methods include:

Diffusion – adding essential oils to a diffuser so their aroma spreads throughout the room.
Topical application – applying diluted essential oils to the skin using a carrier oil.
Baths – adding diluted oils to bath water to promote relaxation.
Massage – mixing essential oils with carrier oils to create massage blends.

Each method provides a different aromatherapy experience.

How Many Essential Oils Should a Beginner Buy?

Beginners do not need to purchase a large number of oils. Starting with a small selection of versatile oils is usually the best approach.

Some commonly recommended beginner oils include:

- Lavender
- Peppermint
- Lemon
- Tea tree
- Eucalyptus
- Frankincense

These oils can be used in many different blends and recipes.

How Long Do Essential Oils Last?

When stored properly, many essential oils can last several years. Their shelf life depends on the type of oil and how it is stored.

Citrus oils generally have a shorter shelf life, often lasting one to two years. Other oils such as lavender, sandalwood, or frankincense may last much longer.

To preserve essential oils:

- Store them in dark glass bottles
- Keep them away from sunlight and heat
- Close the bottles tightly after use

Proper storage helps maintain the aroma and effectiveness of the oils.

Can Essential Oils Be Used Around Children?

Essential oils can sometimes be used around children, but extra caution is necessary. Children have more sensitive skin and may react differently to essential oils than adults. When using essential oils for children:

- Use lower dilution levels
- Avoid strong oils such as peppermint and eucalyptus for very young children
- Always consult a healthcare professional if unsure

Safety should always be the top priority.

Are Essential Oils Safe for Pets?

Some essential oils may be harmful to pets, especially cats and small animals. Pets are more sensitive to certain plant compounds and strong aromas.

If you use a diffuser in your home, make sure the room is well ventilated and that pets can leave the room if they choose.

If you plan to use essential oils around pets regularly, consult a veterinarian for guidance.

How Should Essential Oils Be Stored?

Proper storage helps maintain the quality of essential oils. Essential oils should be stored:

- In dark glass bottles
- Away from heat and sunlight
- In a cool, dry place
- Out of reach of children and pets

Keeping oils properly stored will help preserve their aroma and effectiveness.

Can Essential Oils Replace Medical Treatment?

Essential oils are best used as a **complementary wellness practice**, not as a replacement for professional medical care.

While they may help support relaxation, comfort, and emotional well-being, they should not be used to diagnose, treat, cure, or prevent medical conditions.

If you have a serious health concern, always consult a qualified healthcare professional.

Final Tips for Using Essential Oils

Essential oils can be a wonderful addition to your daily wellness routine when used thoughtfully and safely. As you continue exploring aromatherapy, keep the following tips in mind.

Start simple.
When beginning your essential oil journey, start with a small collection of versatile oils. Oils such as lavender, peppermint, lemon, and tea tree can be used in many different blends and applications.

Use proper dilution.
Because essential oils are highly concentrated, always dilute them with a carrier oil before applying them to the skin. This helps reduce the risk of irritation and allows the oils to be absorbed more comfortably.

Pay attention to quality.
Choose high-quality essential oils from reputable suppliers. Pure essential oils should not contain synthetic fragrances or unnecessary additives.

Experiment with blends.
One of the most enjoyable aspects of aromatherapy is experimenting with different combinations of oils. Over time, you will discover which scents and blends work best for you.

Store oils properly.
Keep your essential oils in dark glass bottles and store them in a cool, dry place away from sunlight. Proper storage helps maintain their quality and effectiveness.

Listen to your body.
Everyone reacts differently to aromas and essential oils. If an oil causes irritation or discomfort, discontinue use and try a different blend.

With a little practice and knowledge, essential oils can become a valuable tool for supporting relaxation, emotional balance, and overall well-being.

Conclusion

Hopefully, by now you have discovered that essential oils can be a simple and enjoyable way to support your health, emotional well-being, and beauty routines. Aromatherapy does not need to be complicated, and with a little knowledge, you can begin incorporating essential oils into your everyday life.

The recipes and examples in this book are intended for common, everyday situations. Essential oils can be a helpful complement to a healthy lifestyle, but they should not replace professional medical advice. If you have a serious health condition, always consult your doctor or a qualified healthcare professional before using essential oils.

Thank you for taking the time to read this book and explore the world of aromatherapy. I hope the information and recipes included here help you feel more confident using essential oils safely and effectively.

If you experience any problems with the printing or delivery of your book, please contact Amazon customer support so they can assist you.

Thank you again for your time, and I wish you success and enjoyment on your journey with essential oils

Katey Lyon
https://www.healthylivingeasy.com/

A Quick Favor Before You Go

If you enjoyed this book and found the information helpful, I would greatly appreciate it if you could take a moment to leave a review on Amazon.

Reviews help other readers discover books that may be useful to them, and they also help authors continue creating helpful content.

Even a short review sharing your thoughts or experience with the book can make a big difference.

Thank you again for taking the time to read this book and for your support.

About the Author

Katey Lyon is the author of several practical guides focused on health, wellness, mindfulness, and personal development. Her books aim to provide simple and easy-to-understand strategies that readers can apply in their everyday lives.

In addition to wellness guides, she has also written journals and workbooks designed to support mindfulness, emotional well-being, and personal growth.

Through her books, Katey's goal is to help readers build healthier habits and create positive lifestyle changes.

Other Books By Katey Lyon

Thank you for reading this book. If you enjoyed learning about essential oils and natural wellness, you may also be interested in exploring some of my other books.

My goal as an author is to create practical guides that help readers improve their daily lives using simple and natural methods. Many of my books focus on topics such as health, wellness, self-improvement, and lifestyle strategies that are easy to understand and apply.

If you found this book helpful, I invite you to take a look at my other titles, where you will discover additional tips, guides, and resources designed to support your personal well-being.

You can find these books on Amazon by searching for **Katey Lyon**.

Thank you again for your support and for taking the time to read my work.

Chakras for Beginners

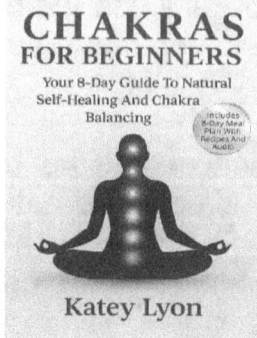

An approachable 8-day guide to natural self-healing and chakra balancing practices.

Meditation for Anxiety and Stress Relief

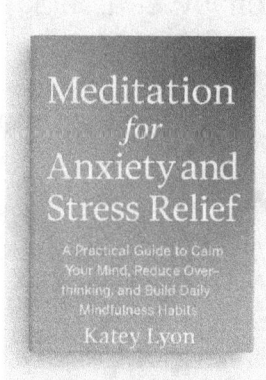

A practical guide to calming the mind, reducing overthinking, and building daily mindfulness habits.

The Mindful Meditation Journal

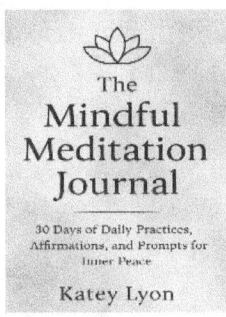

A 30-day guided journal designed to support calm, clarity, and consistent mindfulness practice.

The 5-Minute Gratitude Journal

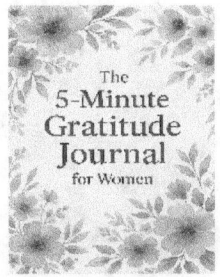

Simple daily prompts designed to build positivity, mindfulness, and emotional balance.

Food, Mood & Exercise Journal

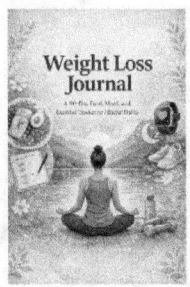

A 90-day tracker designed to build awareness around eating patterns, movement, and emotional triggers.

Emotional Eating Workbook

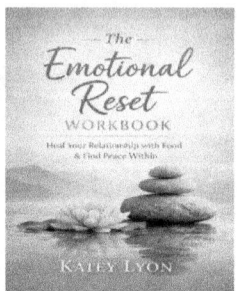

Practical reflection prompts and exercises to help you rebuild your relationship with food and stop starting over.

How to Overcome Jealousy in Relationships

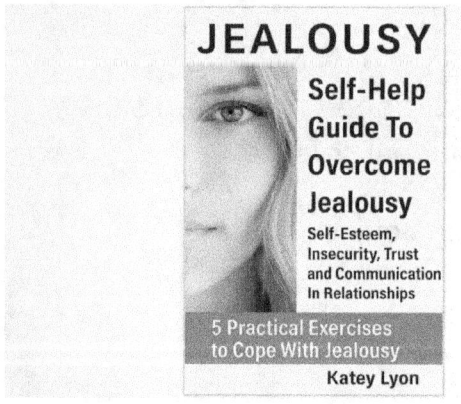

A Practical Self-Help Guide to Building Self-Esteem, Trust, and Emotional Security. If you're wondering how to overcome jealousy in relationships

The Financial Mindset Blueprint

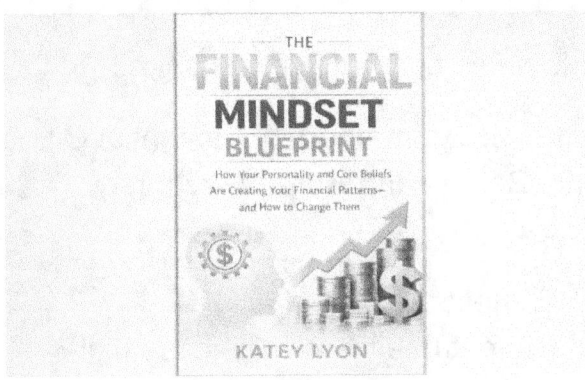

How Your Personality and Core Beliefs Are Creating Your
Financial Patterns — and How to Change Them

References

Essential oil www.britannica.com/topic/essential-oil

Falsetto Sharon, Authentic Aromatherapy. Essential Oils and Blends for Health, Beauty and Home. Skyhorse Publishing. 2014

Essential Oils Health Benefits: https://www.organicfacts.net/health-benefits/essential-oils/pine-essential-oil.html

Canadian Federatio n of Aromatherapists. http://cfacanada.com/aromatherapy/

Acupressure points to treat digestive problems. http://www.modernreflexology.com/acupressure-points-to-treat-digestive-problems/

Price Len, Aromatherapy for health professionals. Churchill Livingstone Elsevier. 2007

3 Ways to Use Aromatherapy to Heal | The Chopra Center. (n.d.). Retrieved from http://www.chopra.com/ccl/3-ways-to-use-aromatherapy-to-heal

Sacred Ascension - Key of Life - Secrets of the Universe. (n.d.). Retrieved from https://sacredascensionmerkaba.com/2016/03/13/urgent-rainbow-portal-31416-32016-

Herb of the Month: Rose | The Oz Blog. (n.d.). Retrieved from http://blog.doctoroz.com/oz-experts/herb-of-the-month-rose

What is some causes of not being able to sleep well ... (n.d.). Retrieved from http://www.medicalquestionsanswers.org/insomnia/what-is-some-causes-of-not-being

Why You Keep Waking Up In The Middle Of The Night." Insert Name of Site in Italics. N.p., n.d. Web. 02 May. 2016 <http://www.huffingtonpost.com/2013/05/30/wake-up-in-the-middle-of-the-night-midd>.

Introduction to Aromatherapy | Health Mastery Systems. (n.d.). Retrieved from http://www.kgstiles.com/aromatherapycourse07_class7_444/

Ratios for Blending Essential Oils – A Reminder of the Basics. (n.d.). Retrieved from https://suzannerbanks.wordpress.com/2014/07/28/ratios-for-blending-essential-oil

Types of Essential Oil Diffusers - Welledia. (n.d.). Retrieved from http://welledia.com/blogs/aromablog/34891521-types-of-essential-oil-diffusers

Health pick-Pathways for entry. (n.d.). Retrieved from http://healthepic.com/aroma/static/how-oils-enter-the-body.htm

Aromatherapy « Canadian Federation of
Aromatherapists. (n.d.). Retrieved from
http://cfacanada.com/aromatherapy/

aromatherapy | Britannica.com. (n.d.). Retrieved from
http://www.britannica.com/topic/aromatherapy

Essential Oils | Vibrant Life Aromatherapy | Derbyshire.
(n.d.). Retrieved from
http://www.vibrantlifearomatherapy.co.uk/essential-oils/

Holistic and therapeutic massage | Herbs and Hands.
(n.d.). Retrieved from http://herbsandhands.co.uk/holistic-
and-therapeutic-massage/